PRACTICAL WELLNESS

PRACTICAL WELLNESS·

A Guide To Empowering Choices In Your Health and Well-being

Laurie Neri Barrett

ISBN-13: 9781978024632
ISBN-10: 1978024630
Library of Congress Control Number: 2017915787
CreateSpace Independent Publishing Platform
North Charleston, South Carolina

This book is dedicated to the memory of Karen Lopez Bartlett, nurse practitioner, for sharing her passion in integrative medicine with me and all whom she touched. Her dedication to creating awareness in the health and wellness industry will forever remain in my heart. I believe that without her guidance from the spirit realm, this book would have not been possible. Even though she is not seen, her work is still in progress. Thank you, Karen, in much love and light.

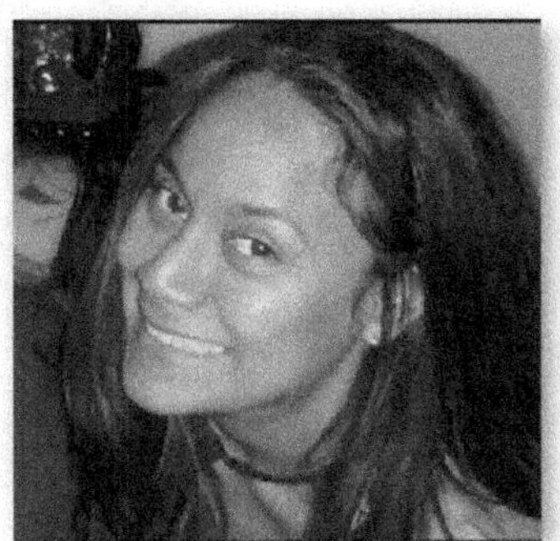

Karen Lopez Bartlett

Contents

Acknowledgment of Gratitude

I don't believe I have enough time to put into words how grateful I am for every day of my life and for the love from God and all who assist me from the spirit realm daily. The wounds in my life brought me a gift in spiritual growth and the knowledge to serve those around me.

I recently had a dear friend send me a Papyrus greeting card with this beautiful message in it: "Legends say that hummingbirds float free of time carrying our hopes for love, joy, and celebration. The hummingbird's delicate grace reminds us that life is rich, beauty is everywhere, every personal connection has meaning, and laughter is life's sweetest creation." Each time I read this, my soul is filled with emotion.

For my loving husband, who has graciously supported, assisted, and allowed me to follow the path I have chosen. How thankful I am for his trust and picking up the pieces in life when I could not.

For my son, who tells me frequently throughout the day how much he loves me. This is his way, I believe, of bringing me back in the moment.

For my mother, the woman who has taught me how to love, forgive, and be generous to others with all I have been blessed with. And my father, his life showed me how to be fearless when moving forward with any goal.

And last but certainly not least, for my furry babies. They teach me each day to ground in love and to believe in myself, and they give me the opportunity to experience receiving the greatest gift of all—unconditional love.

Introduction

If you don't take care of your body, where are you going to live?

—UNKNOWN

Your remarkable body!

After thirty years in the health, fitness, and wellness business, I've found there is not much in this realm I have not experienced within my own body and spirit *or* had the opportunity to assist clients with on their path. It has been and will continue to be a lifelong journey of learning and shifting. As we all know, the only thing constant in life is change. It is all in the moment. What is good for you today probably will not be so in three months.

In the beginning of my career, it was all about how a person looked. Now it has evolved to how a person feels. Not just for my clients but also for myself. The world of fitness has evolved with the changing needs of our population. It is now about function before beauty, as it should be for any age. You wouldn't build a house on a poor foundation. It may work for a while—even look good. But at some point, that home will crumble. Just like your body—the home in which your spirit resides. Even though I'm the paid teacher, I can say that I frequently feel like the student. Clients will bring issues that force me to continue to challenge the depth of my knowledge on many levels. But more than that, life has brought me many of my own wounds that I have chosen to learn how to heal and to teach others about. I realized that if I want to change the world, I have to heal and better myself. That is where shift begins.

As a bodyworker, I can say that there are no two of us the same. Our beliefs, problems, and worries and how we each manifest these in our physical body are always unique. I am constantly reminding myself what Jan Engels-Smith, author of *Through the Rabbit Hole* said. "We are a Soul/Spirit having a human experience." When we begin to nurture the heart and soul, our entire health will improve. While I am not here to critique or judge an individual's choices in life, my mission is to offer suggestions on the many remedies available to hopefully make our time here a bit easier. When I work with people either in movement or massage, I am always mindful of what my choices are to assist them on their path of healing—not necessarily with words but always with intent. I am frequently asked for my advice and guidance on many health and wellness issues. That is why I have been guided to write this book.

As a working mom over fifty, I know that the stress, anxiety, and many shifts in my body are shared with others in my age group. We are all searching for assistance to feel better and to function better physically, mentally, emotionally, and spiritually. And, well, maybe even look better!

Chapter One
Myofascial Release

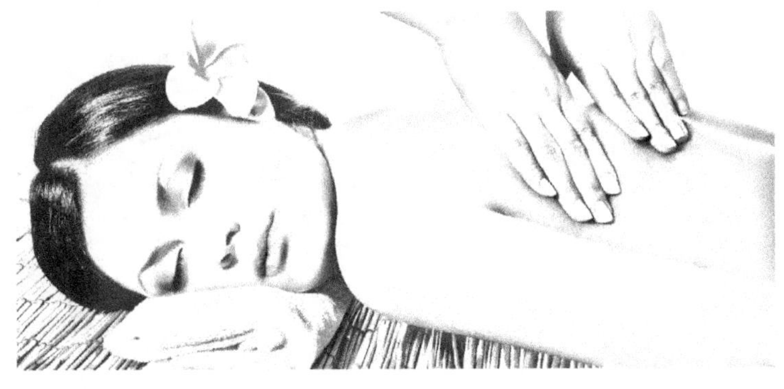

Myofascial Release

The way to health is to have an aromatic bath and a scented massage every day.

—HIPPOCRATES

There is no way I could write about all the types of bodywork available to each of us in just one chapter. That would be its own book. I have listed some of the more common body therapies that I believe would be beneficial to be familiar with. Massage coupled with a good movement program work toward long-term goals.

MASSAGE THERAPY

Love is a fruit in season at all times, and within reach of every hand.

—MOTHER TERESA

Therapeutic massage provides stress reduction, deep relaxation, increased circulation, and relief from physical pain. It stimulates the lymphatic system, which will flush out toxins and excess water from the body, thereby improving your immune system.

Here is some advice about both choosing a therapist for yourself and receiving a true therapeutic massage. First and foremost, deeper is not always better. If you are in pain while receiving a massage, there is no benefit to letting go on any level. Applying appropriate pressure without pain is essential to allowing you and your nervous system to release. A knowledgeable and intuitive therapist knows what techniques to do and how deep to work. Do not get caught up with labeling. Sometimes it's just a spa's creative way to charge you more.

Remember, ultimately you and your spirit are the healer. A good therapist knows this. Having textbook knowledge is important, but so is knowledge from a higher source—intuition—which is God and spirit speaking to me during the session. I always offer a prayer of guidance to help bring healing to the client where it is most needed.

FOAM ROLLING

The use of a foam roller is essential to your wellness program. There is nothing better for self-myofascial release. It's always available any time of the day. Rolling before your workouts will increase blood flow and decrease your chance of injury. Your connective tissue (fascia) connects each body part to the next. Unfortunately, from injury, improper movement patterns, and poor hydration, the muscles don't glide efficiently through movement. What do you suppose happens if you begin your training session loading this hot mess?

The more you roll, the more harmoniously it will all start to work. Quality of movement is always the goal. The more muscles we wake up and invite to the party, the less pain and injury we will experience.

YAMUNA BODY ROLLING

A woman by the name of Yamuna Zake created this approach to self-massage. Classes are taught by certified teachers utilizing different-sized balls with various pressures appropriate for your body. This system serves as a self-healing tool on many levels. In addition to releasing physical restrictions, there is nerve-root stimulation along the spine, which can be great for stimulating organ function and overall circulation. Foot wakers are one of my favorite products. This great tool can bring blood flow and circulation and help make your feet more flexible, which in turn will create more range of motion. Your feet are the foundation of your body. How you take in energy from the ground up is critical to all your moving parts.

The best part about Yamuna body rolling and the foam roller is that you are in charge of pressure, frequency, and the ability to maintain your body whenever and wherever you are. I use my Yamuna ball regularly. There are some areas of the body that no other tool can access like the Yamuna ball.

ACTIVE RELEASE TECHNIQUE (ART)

ART was started over thirty years ago by Dr. P. Michael Leahy, a chiropractic sports physician. ART is a patented state-of-the-art soft-tissue technique that moves the body while massaging the injured area. The goal is to break down adhesions in order to restore normal range of motion, strength, and function within muscles, tendons, ligaments, and nerves.

When an injury has been with you a long time and it is not getting better, this is a great treatment to receive. As a massage therapist, I can say that a good ART practitioner will be able to break down that scar tissue in fewer sessions than I ever could.

My body is my machine. If I want to support myself and my family, I do not have the luxury of taking time off. And for that matter, who does? ART has got and will continue to get me the quality of movement I want to continue to live my life.

ROLFING

Ida Rolf, PhD, is recognized as the pioneer in soft-tissue manipulation and movement education. Both her and her family's health problems are what drove her to experiment with many forms of alternative healing methods. Her studies led her to believe that anatomical structure, alignment, and physiologic function are at the core of many modalities of healing. I can't help but think about how much less stress there is on all our organs when our structural body is working properly and allowing the force of gravity to flow through it.

She developed a program of ten sessions to be given in a specific order. Rolfing focuses on improving how the entire structural body aligns. Each session progresses from the previous session and prepares the systems of the body to receive the next treatment. For example, if your neck always hurts even after receiving a massage, there could be something in another area of the body restricting a complete release. These sessions should be followed by, of course, a movement program to assist the body in continuing to improve and hold alignment.

She passed away in 1979 at the age of eighty-three. The Rolfing Institute of Structural Integration continues her work certifying practitioners. There are close to two thousand practitioners worldwide. I would say, "Brilliant. Job well done, Ida Rolf."

ASTON PATTERNING

Aston Patterning techniques were developed by dancer and massage therapist Judith Aston, BA, MFA Pilates. She taught classes at a community college focusing on posture awareness and movement patterns.

Judith was led to Dr. Ida Rolf after two consecutive car accidents. Traditional treatment got her only so far. She saw dramatic changes for the better in her body after Rolfing. In 1968, she was asked by Dr. Rolf to design a movement program to be taught to both Rolfers and recipients of Rolfing. They believed that structural bodywork had to be coupled with a movement program to make a significant change.

After five years of teaching this program, it evolved. Aston's work includes movement education, fitness training, ergonomic modification, and massage. She believes that movement occurs in three-dimensional and asymmetrical spirals. This not only corrected muscular imbalances but also helped develop your body awareness with the environment around you. As Rolfers learned to move with more ease and less tension, they began to notice that the bodywork they were giving was also gentler for both them and their clients. This realization that practitioners who used their bodies correctly would not impose the tension in their bodies to those of their clients is what makes the Aston paradigm different from Rolfing.

I have had the opportunity to work with an Aston practitioner. There are not a great number of practitioners as the training takes a great commitment of time. I took one course in this extensive training. That four days changed how I looked at the body—even how to prop your body while sleeping in different positions. This is phenomenal work. Watching an Aston practitioner at work (and receiving work from one) is an amazing experience. They see things in movement that the average trained eye does not.

DRY NEEDLING

Nothing can reach the depths of soft-tissue dysfunction like dry needling. I know I would have been in surgery a long time ago without the help of this amazing treatment.

It is a Western form of acupuncture based on the study of neuro-anatomy, the musculoskeletal and nervous system. Dry needling is usually performed by physical therapists and chiropractors but also by medical doctors. Both dry needling and traditional Eastern acupuncture use the same needles, but dry needling treats musculoskeletal pain rather than energetic meridians.

Dr. Janet Travell was one of the pioneers of this but not with dry needles. She used procaine (a local numbing anesthetic) injections with vapocoolant sprays to relieve pain before injections. These sprays are still popular in sports medicine today. Her experience treating musculoskeletal pain led her to the White House. She treated John F. Kennedy, who suffered back pain from injuries from World War II. She wrote a book along with David Simons called *Myofascial Pain and Dysfunction: The Trigger Point Manual.* This was the first book recommended for me to buy when I was in massage school. My head was in that book from the beginning of my massage career. Even though massages help tremendously, my elbow was never going to reach the depths of a needle.

Everyone feels this treatment differently. Personally, I feel immediately better followed by soreness the next day. By the second or third day, I feel a significant improvement.

GRASTON TECHNIQUE

The Graston technique treats scar tissue and fascial restrictions using various specially designed, stainless-steel instruments. They look like surgical tools. Even though they are not surgical instruments, I am quite sure these tools can be very dangerous if treatment is given by an untrained individual.

The patient benefits are a faster recovery, increased range of motion, and a possible reduction of the need to take anti-inflammatory medications.

There are more than twenty-four thousand clinicians worldwide. Physical therapists, chiropractors, and athletic trainers are the main providers of this technique. Graston-certified individuals go through quite an extensive training program, which is consistently updated to reflect the latest research in rehabilitation. My holistic vet, who specializes in chiropractic and soft-tissue manipulation, uses these instruments on my pets also.

Having received this treatment, I highly recommend it. The instrument glides over the adhesions underneath the skin. Although it has never been uncomfortable for me to receive, the clinician can adjust the intensity to the appropriate tolerance level of the patient. As usual this treatment should be followed by rehabilitative exercises.

MUSCLE ACTIVATION TECHNIQUE (MAT)

Even though this is not a myofascial treatment, you are on the table fully clothed while receiving the treatment. MAT opens the channels of communication from brain to muscle. It is a noninvasive approach, in which the practitioner evaluates which muscles are or are not contracting by assessing range of motion. Loss of muscle contraction can lead to limited range of motion and joint instability.

You might say it's a jump start to get your muscles working again. This approach is used on muscles that have not worked in a while due to injury or inactivity. Precise force is applied to activate muscles to work efficiently again.

A massage license is not required to be a MAT practitioner. When choosing someone, I believe it is important that the person have an extensive background in rehabilitative movement.

Chapter Two
Fitness and Movement

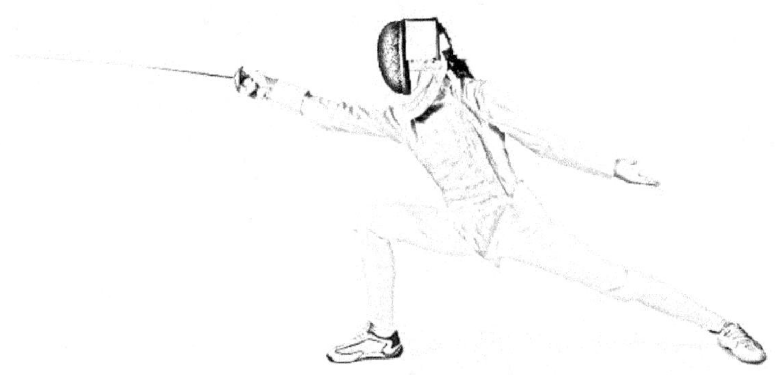

2

Fitness and Movement

Move well, move often.

—GRAY COOK

This chapter will discuss various types of exercise for function, stability, strength, mobility, and relaxation. These five qualities all offer great benefits to our overall health. I have covered some of the movement therapies popular to many people either from participation or simply having read about. By no means does your exercise program stop with what I have discussed below. Each form of movement I have listed will help you decide what type of exercise is appropriate to perform and when it would be beneficial to your current needs.

THE FUNCTIONAL MOVEMENT SCREEN (FMS)

The FMS is based on seven fundamental movements. It is an objective tool to determine if someone's movement patterns are optimal, acceptable, or dysfunctional. A score is generated, and specific exercises are customized for each individual. This provides great simplicity and feedback for the client and professional, both in the initial screen and future screens after client has been working on imbalances. The screen will identify asymmetry and dysfunction, which is said to increase risk of injury by three-and-one-half times.

Gray Cook and Lee Burton created this system. This philosophy is not only based on current science and research but also draws on an artistic and visionary side. As each client is unique in every experience of life, coaches and trainers must be willing to view the client through many different eyes. It is evident in the corrective-movement program that proceeds the screen that they have studied and practiced many of the exercise programs I will discuss below, such as the importance of breathing from yoga and full-body cooperative movement based on the Feldenkrais method.

The FMS is used by many reputable organizations, such as the NFL, NBA, MLB, NCAA, and US military, to name a few. As a personal trainer, I think it's my favorite tool in the box. It takes all the guess work out of where the weak link is in the body, and it gives me a great baseline for programming sessions. Most important, it assures clients that they are headed in the right direction to feeling better. After all, isn't that what they are paying me to do?

THE FUNCTIONALLY FIT BODY

To enjoy the glow of good health, you must exercise.

—GENE TUNNEY

If you are currently involved in an exercise program, I believe your questions would be, "Am I benefiting from my current routine, and am I exercising properly and efficiently?"

Usually by the time someone has sought me out for my services, there is frustration at some level that something in the person's body is not working correctly. Most times it is pain somewhere in the body, and it has been there for quite a while. No amount of weight training, golfing, or running seems to improve it, and these activities are not going to.

There must be a balance in the body between mobility, stability, and strength. Somewhere along the way—usually with injuries, inactivity, trauma and so on—our body figures out a new way to move outside of our primal movement patterns we instinctively knew as infants. So even though we feel as though we have healed through our injuries, most times we have healed around them. The body and mind are very smart. You will figure out a whole new way to move to avoid pain.

The result is shutting down certain muscles and overcompensating with others.

A few years back, I had a girl referred to me by a client. Her complaint was extreme tightness in her calves when squatting. She attended CrossFit three times a week. After screening her, I explained to her what was going on and gave her corrective exercises to assist this imbalance. I also told her that it would be a good idea to back off CrossFit for a while until this imbalance improved. I guess she didn't like my advice, because she never came back. Please understand that you cannot build strength on top of dysfunction. Adding more weight to her squat will only make her a stronger, more dysfunctional squatter. I am sure her imbalance was present long before performing CrossFit.

If you don't listen to the warning signs in your physical body, it *will* stop you. And it may not be pretty. Backing off and slowing down for a while are better than being told to stop your favorite activity forever because you are beyond repair.

When you are searching for an answer to truly being fit, ask yourself this question: "Am I functioning in my daily life tasks as well as I would like?" If not, the amount of weight you are pushing in the gym does not matter; it is only a meaningless number in your head.

THE ORDER OF COMMAND

In all my years as a fitness professional, the most common complaint brought to me from clients is, "My hamstrings and lower back are always tight." I wish I could tell you that stretching on its own would correct this problem, but that is just a small fraction of the imbalance.

Tight hamstrings and lower back are caused by the transversus abdominis (TA), multifidus, and the glutes not firing properly. If this chain of command is not in order, then your hamstrings and lower back are doing a job they were not hired to perform.

When our bodies begin to move, the core muscles *should be* the first to activate. Usually injuries and negative habitual-movement patterns prevent this from happening.

If you create good pelvic stabilization, your torso and legs can easily transfer energy to support efficient muscular engagement so that your back, hamstrings, and joints do not have to overwork.

Your core is your foundation of strength. The TA and multifidus are engaged through the neutral spine only, which happens when lying supine or prone, kneeling, half kneeling, hands and knees (quadruped), and standing. This is not to be confused with the overworked rectus abdominis, which is a superficial muscle providing no pelvic stabilization whatsoever. If you are performing abdominal crunches in your current exercise program, you are working the rectus abdominis. This certainly will not contribute to your long-term goals.

Next in command are the glutes. Big muscle, big job. Sitting, driving, and poor training will force the hip-flexor muscles to work instead of the glutes. Are you starting to see the pattern of pain?

When hiring a trainer, be sure that you are working with someone who is qualified in recognizing these imbalances and knows the way to retrain negative patterns of movement with the proper exercises, myofascial work utilizing the foam roller, or other techniques suggested in my previous chapter. And of utmost importance, the trainer must train you in body movement, not just body parts.

PILATES EXERCISE

> *To achieve the highest accomplishments within the scope of our capabilities in all walks of life, we must constantly strive to acquire strong, healthy bodies and develop our minds to the limits of our ability.*

> —JOSEPH PILATES

Evolved from techniques created by Joseph H. Pilates more than eighty years ago, Pilates exercise improves strength, flexibility, balance, coordination, and posture. It creates strong abdominals, glutes, and back. It's gentle enough for mothers-to-be yet challenging enough for athletes and super fit individuals. It's a program that can work for everyone, regardless of age or condition.

However, all these benefits totally depend on *who* is teaching you. First and foremost, it is all about finding the neutral spine. That is where all the benefits come from in any form of movement, not just Pilates.

Footwork, leg circles, frogs, and so on have no benefit to you if you are not coached properly from someone who has a good eye for whether you are holding proper core alignment. Range of motion in all movement should match your ability in your core strength level. For example, why are you aiming for big, large leg circles when you are arching your back and doming your belly throughout the movement? I hate to tell you this, but you are causing more harm than good. Smaller movement equals more stability.

Time and time again, I see Pilates teachers too concerned about showing all the great choreography progressions and taking students to the next level of difficult movement when they are not ready. And they may never be. This is sometimes due to lack of experience or the provider they have trained under.

If you are in the market for private sessions, be sure to look for someone who preferably has an extensive fitness or rehabilitation background as well as Pilates and who does not give you the cookie-cutter workout. That is not what you are paying for in a private session. If classes are your choice, it might be a good idea to take a couple of private sessions first to get your fundamentals strong.

THE FELDENKRAIS METHOD

Lotion is motion, and rest is rust.

—Nicholas A. DiNubile, MD

I cannot say how very much I respect this approach to well-being. The Feldenkrais method, developed by Moshe Feldenkrais, is based on the principles of physics, physiology, and neurology.

A Feldenkrais practitioner will direct his or her attention to movements that appear to be difficult or inefficient and will teach slow, repetitive movement sequences to bring awareness to all parts of self. The beauty of this therapy is that you progress gradually at your own pace, utilizing your body's innate wisdom. Imagine your entire body cooperating harmoniously when you move.

Feldenkrais is not a substitute for exercise. It is meant to enhance other forms of exercise. The goal is to improve overall performance.

Moshe Feldenkrais developed what we know today as the foam roller. However, his version was made from wood. He never patented his idea. Too bad, right?

YOGA

Above all, learn how to breathe correctly.

True flexibility can be achieved only when all muscles are uniformly developed.

—Joseph Pilates

There are so many benefits from yoga. The most important is breath. If you get nothing else but that, you are leaps and bounds ahead. Your lungs are about how you take in life. It is the first breath of air that introduces you to the earth.

Learning to breathe calms the nervous system. This results in better sleep, less muscular tension, better digestion, and a more balanced endocrine system. When clients have neck issues, one of the first things I usually find is that they are shallow breathers. This can cause a whole chain of side effects, such as dizziness or lightheadedness and headaches. Coaching the breath out of the shoulders and chest along with a proper movement program will get great results.

I recently had a client come to me complaining about tight hamstrings and lower back. She told me she had been doing yoga for fifteen years. When I asked her if she had seen any improvement over the years, she said, "No, not for more than a couple of hours. But my teacher says if I stick with it, it will change."

What? I told her that yoga alone was not going to fix this problem because she had no lumbopelvic stabilization. I also told her that if she worked on this imbalance, I was confident that her yoga would also improve.

Also, every pose is not for every body. For example, in the above case, forward bending with straight legs is a nightmare waiting to happen. If you have injuries that require rehabilitation, it may be necessary to put your yoga on hold until you are released from the doctor or told by a physical therapist what is safe for your body to perform.

Chapter Three

Organ Function and the Endocrine System

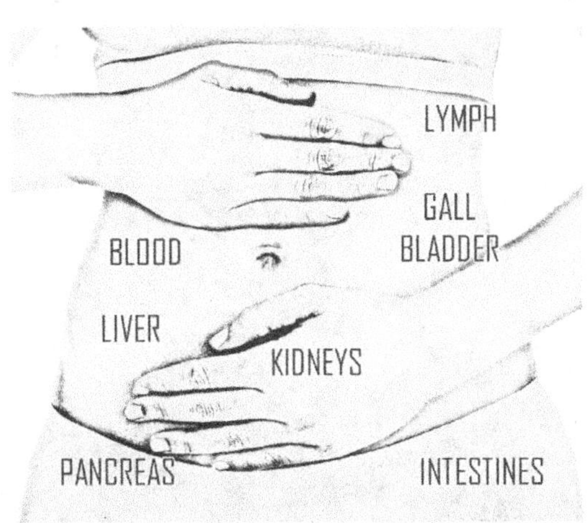

3

Organ Function and the Endocrine System

The art of healing comes from nature, not from the physician.
Therefore, the physician must start from nature, with an open
mind.

—PARACELSUS

Before I begin this chapter, I want to stress the importance of finding a health-care provider who practices integrative medicine, someone who has a great appreciation for both Western and Eastern medicine. If you are currently taking any medications, a medical doctor or nurse practitioner will understand how natural treatments mix with medications. You may always need your medications, but it may be possible to wean you off them or cut dosages down with natural forms of treatment.

Compounded medications, such as thyroid medications and hormone-replacement therapy, will require a prescription from a knowledgeable medical professional. Do not self-diagnose or self-treat.

GALLBLADDER AND LIVER

For every minute you remain angry, you give up sixty seconds of
peace of mind.

—RALPH WALDO EMERSON

The gallbladder is a small, sack-like organ in the upper right of the abdomen. It is located on the right side below the rib cage. The liver sits above it. The gallbladder, liver, and pancreas make up what is called the biliary system in our body. The biliary system produces bile. Bile is made in the liver along with enzymes, and it aids in digestion of fats and cholesterol. Bile is stored in our gallbladder. When we eat, the gallbladder contracts and pushes bile into our small intestines so that our body can begin to excrete fat-soluble toxins out of the body and begin to assist our overall digestive system to absorb fats.

Gallstones become present when the body is trying to detoxify an overabundance of cholesterol in the liver. There are many cleanses to assist the relaxing of the bile duct in order to allow these excessive amounts of cholesterol and small stones to pass. However, a medical emergency can exist if a stone becomes lodged anywhere in the bile-duct system. This will most likely result in a gallbladder removal. If you have been diagnosed as having gallstones, please do not perform any type of cleanse without the guidance of a qualified integrative health doctor. An ultrasound may be required first to be sure stones are not too large and calcified to pass through the common bile duct.

Most doctors don't think it's a big deal to remove the gallbladder because the liver can just take over. Without the gallbladder, there is nothing to tell the liver *when* to do its job. The gallbladder is the decision maker. Not having a gallbladder leads to an overworked liver and a body with constant diarrhea. That doesn't sound like fun in my book of life.

What are signs that your gallbladder and liver are not functioning at an optimal level? My favorite symptoms that everyone ignores are heartburn and indigestion. Others are right-side abdominal pain, which may also be painful under the shoulder blade, stomach pain after eating, especially greasy food, and discolored stool.

As I mentioned earlier, there are many cleanses for the gallbladder and liver. This is an easy flush. Five days before the flush, drink two quarts of apple juice per day or six apples combined with one tablespoon of raw apple-cider vinegar in water three times throughout the day. If you cannot tolerate that many apples or that much juice, a malic-acid supplement may be taken. Malic acid, which is present in apples, will soften your gallstones. But apples also have pectin in them, which will push more old bile out and force the liver to produce new bile to clean the biliary system. It is also a good idea to eat more vegetables, fruits, and nuts for the week.

On the fifth day, eat one grapefruit and drink a bottle of magnesium citrate for dinner. (Yum!) At bedtime drink one-half cup of olive oil mixed with one-third cup of freshly squeezed lemon juice. I use a straw and push way in the back of my throat to get this combination down. Go to bed lying on your right side with your knees pulled toward your chest.

You will have many bowel movements; the ones closest to morning are where all the action hits. My first flush was shocking. I could not believe all the small stones I passed. Stones will float and have a sand-like texture. They can be the size of a seed or a cherry pit. Some people like to repeat this cleanse again in a few weeks. If you are thirty or older and this is your first time, it is probably a good idea to repeat this flush. I perform this flush yearly. It has never been a repeat of the first. But I drink apple-cider vinegar daily and eat well.

In traditional Chinese medicine, the hours of eleven at night to one in the morning represent gallbladder function. Are you waking up between these hours? As with the physical, there is always an emotional manifestation. Possibly you are having trouble making decisions in your life. If you are waking up between these hours on a regular basis, this can deplete your gallbladder's energy stores.

It's almost impossible to separate the gallbladder from the liver. The liver is your largest organ, and what a tough job it has. Everything you eat, drink, and breath is processed, eliminated, or stored for later use. It is impossible to have sufficient energy, good circulation, healthy digestion and metabolism, a strong immune system, and balanced hormones with an overburdened liver.

Let's review what we put in our bodies in our "civilized" world: alcohol, sugar, medications, artificial sweeteners, and acetaminophen, not to mention the air we breathe. All the above on a regular basis can overwhelm this organ. If you take care of the gallbladder, the liver gets help, too. There are many herbal supplements for the liver. I don't recommend using any of them without a qualified professional. You are trying to cleanse it, not stress it out more than it already is. It all starts with your base diet. As Hippocrates said, "The greatest medicine of all is teach people how not to need it." I believe this applies to not only pharmaceuticals but also to herbal treatments.

The hours of one to three in the morning represent the liver. If you are awake at this time, this could be a sign that an imbalance is present. Symptoms, can result in headaches, fatigue, anemia, and, for women, irregular cycles. Ask yourself, "What am I holding on to? What may I be angry about?"

In the upcoming chapter "Alternative Remedies," I will further discuss how I believe acupuncture, colonics, and castor-oil packs can balance, purify, and assist physical and emotional release for these ever-so-important organs.

APPENDIX

If you listen to the Western medicine community, they will tell you that the appendix is a useless organ that we do not need. I'm pretty sure God didn't put it there to fill up space. One's experience with the appendix is usually a bad one: either appendicitis or removal. But what went wrong? Why did it happen? What do you need to know moving forward after it's been removed?

According to Dr. Edward Group III, author of *The Green Body Cleanse*, the appendix is a tube-shaped sac that is located near the juncture of the small and large intestine. It is present in humans and a small number of mammals. Many scientists believe that this organ was once used to assist us in digesting tree bark. Since we don't eat tree bark anymore (maybe we should), it is said that we no longer need it. But let's not jump to conclusions too quickly. Duke University Medical Center has research to enlighten us all a bit more.

Unless you have been living under a rock for years, you will understand the importance of healthy flora and bacteria in our digestive system. When illness or disease strikes the body, it attacks our healthy bacteria. When this happens, our appendix acts as a backup, like a reservoir. As our immune system fights off illness, healthy bacteria reenter the digestive tract from the appendix.

According to studies, lymphoid tissue accumulates in the appendix after birth and helps produce antibodies. Immune-system cells live in the appendix to protect healthy bacteria. I can't stress this enough: it *all* starts in the gut!

Appendicitis is serious business. It may not always end in removal of the organ. Usually appendicitis occurs when there is an obstruction of either food or fecal matter inside the appendix. This blockage will increase pressure and impair blood flow. An infection in the digestive tract can also cause lymph nodes to swell and create pressure on the appendix.

Whether you still have your appendix or not, you must eat fermented foods or take a quality probiotic. Examples of fermented foods are sauerkraut, raw pickles, kombucha tea, kimchi (Asian fermented cabbage), and raw unfiltered vinegar. However, if your appendix has been removed and careful attention is not given to this situation, there could be a very compromised immune system in your future.

HYPOTHYROIDISM

There is so much to write about on this topic in order to clearly understand just how important and critical this gland, the thyroid, is to us in so many ways.

Symptoms of hypothyroidism include fatigue, disturbed sleep, trouble losing weight, intolerance to cold, constipation, poor memory, depression, skin disorders, brittle nails, menstrual problems, hair loss, headaches, infertility, fibrocystic breast disease, ovarian cysts, recurrent infections, chronic yeast infections, and cholesterol issues. Wow, I'm exhausted just listing them all!

Inadequate production of thyroid hormone will lead to other endocrine and glandular dysfunction, such as with the pituitary, ovarian, and adrenal glands. Are you starting to see the domino effect?

How many people do you know, maybe even yourself, who have these symptoms, go to the doctor, and are told they are depressed, need to be on some sort of depression medication, and need to seek psychiatric help? The patient wonders, "Well, am I depressed because I'm tired or tired because I'm depressed?" On an emotional level, thyroid dysfunction is about your "will" to keep moving forward. How can one empower themselves?

This is why most doctors don't believe in chronic fatigue immune dysfunction (CFIDS); they are not educated to treat this, so it is swept under the rug. So many medical conditions can result from lack of proper treatment: anemia, infections, cancer, autoimmune disorders. And guess what? According to David Brownstein, MD, women are affected at a ratio of three to one over men.

I bet by now you are curious, as I was, as to *why* women suffer thyroid dysfunction more than men. Every doctor I went to could never answer this. Then I did my research and found an answer.

THE IODINE CONNECTION

The big question is, why do women have more thyroid issues than men? Due to larger amounts of reproductive tissue, women require *more* iodine to regulate proper hormone synthesis throughout their entire reproductive system. Iodine found in the ovaries is second to the amount found in the thyroid. If your reproductive tissue does not have enough iodine, it will seek it from your thyroid and thus leave you depleted. Our bodies are so smart.

Therefore, so many women suffer from fibrocystic disease, ovarian and uterine cysts, and polycystic ovary syndrome (PCOS). When the ovaries are starved of iodine, it can lead to infertility, miscarriages, and many other issues. It is also linked to autoimmune diseases and inflammation in the body, such as arthritis. Iodine is needed to detoxify the body of mercury, fluorides, chlorides, and bromides, which are all very prominent in many foods and products we ingest.

Compounded desiccated thyroid, or pharmaceutical prescription Armour Thyroid, contains both T4 and T3 hormones. Both of these require a prescription. Desiccated thyroid comes from pigs (porcine). I prefer compounded over prepacked Armour Thyroid. Compounding can get you precise amounts of T4 and T3, which will result in your thyroid functioning more efficiently. Every batch of Armour will differ because it is natural. Selenium and iodine are also needed for T4-to-T3 conversion in the liver. T4 alone is *not* sufficient. Therefore, synthetic thyroid drugs, such as Synthroid and Levothyroxine, do not seem to improve symptoms in most people in the long term.

It is also very common for a person to have all the symptoms of hypothyroidism with a negative blood test. That is because blood tests do not detect what is happening at the deepest level of function in the body, which is cellular. Did your doctor check your levels of iodine in the body? It is possible that sufficient iodine may be all you need to assist the thyroid to function better. How many of you have thinning hair and have been told that your thyroid is normal?

If you have these symptoms and have been told that all is well with your thyroid, I encourage you to do your research and find a qualified doctor who is familiar with the appropriate tests.

ADRENAL GLANDS

The adrenal glands are in the back, located on top of the kidneys. These glands are responsible for many hormones in both men and women. They are the fight-or-flight hormones, such as epinephrine and norepinephrine, that assist us in stressful situations. And then there are the steroid hormones that assist the body in fighting infection. The main hormone is hydrocortisone. This provides our body with glucose and amino acids and regulates blood-sugar metabolism.

Other sex hormones produced in the adrenal glands are DHEA, testosterone, estrogen, progesterone, and pregnenolone. DHEA and testosterone are responsible for muscle and tissue repair and building. Men and women also produce these from testicles and ovaries. As women age, such as during menopause, the ovaries are no longer kicking out anymore hormones, so now our only hope is a bit of something from our adrenals.

Are you starting to see how constantly being stressed makes you fat, tired, and sick all the time? First you produce too much hydrocortisone, and then you hit depletion. Now let's add aging, such as menopause. There is no need to wonder anymore why you have belly fat and depression. There are many other diseases—such as diabetes, high cholesterol, and thyroid and autoimmune disorders—that result after long-term adrenal imbalance.

So many people have low blood pressure. This can sometimes be linked to some sort of imbalance in adrenal hormones.

HYDROCORTISONE

Hydrocortisone is a hormone produced in the adrenal glands. Without sufficient levels of this hormone, the body's ability to handle stressful situations becomes depleted. This includes fighting infections and illness. If you are constantly getting sick, one cold after another, with longer-than-normal recovery times and constant exhaustion, you may be low in hydrocortisone.

The body produces about forty milligrams of hydrocortisone a day from the adrenal glands. When a person is deficient in this, physiologic doses of ten to twenty milligrams will allow the person's adrenals to begin to function again.

About a year after giving birth to my son, I knew that something was not functioning well in my body. I went to a clinical nutritionist, who gave me a saliva test. I collected my saliva four times in one day, as the adrenal glands surge hormone four times daily. When the lab results came back, I was in full-blown adrenal exhaustion. No wonder all I wanted to do was sleep. I also could not lose my last five pounds of baby weight. I was then referred to a physician for treatment. Hydrocortisone was prescribed for me to take three times daily, coordinated with the times our bodies produce hydrocortisone.

My reading session at eleven at night was the only time my body was producing sufficient hormone. Of course, that is when the least amount is needed in our day. In addition to hydrocortisone, DHEA, in the amount of ten milligrams per day, and specific B vitamins (B5 and B6) were also given. After three months, I gradually cut my dose of hydrocortisone, and doses of DHEA along with B vitamins continued. In three months, I felt great, *and* I lost all my weight.

High stress levels will deplete your body of B vitamins. They are essential to adrenal function as well as to your nervous system. I will discuss this further in the nutrition chapter. (It can get complicated.)

I believe that imbalanced adrenals may be the precursor to thyroid problems. If only our Western medical world addressed these issues, there might just be less thyroid disease. There are medical doctors who do treat the endocrine system in its entirety. A good health practitioner can get you back on track and keep your energy good, your weight balanced, and hopefully your sleep sufficient.

DEHYDROEPIANDROSTERONE (DHEA)

DHEA is a hormone produced in the adrenal glands. When the body is low in DHEA, the body's ability to fight infection decreases. This includes diseases like autoimmune disorders, asthma, high cholesterol, diabetes, cardiovascular disease, hypertension, osteoporosis, allergies, depression, Alzheimer's, and, yes, even cancer.

DHEA is converted in the body to other hormones, such as testosterone, estrogen, and progesterone. Supplementation can help with muscle mass, fatigue, better skin, and the above-mentioned problems. When DHEA is given to premenopausal women, it will usually bring their estrogen and progesterone levels back in balance.

Even though DHEA can be bought over the counter, it should be monitored by a qualified professional. Small, clinical dosages are recommended based on specific testing.

PREGNENOLONE

Pregnenolone is a steroid hormone produced from cholesterol in the adrenal glands. The best way to think of this hormone is that it is the first one off the conveyor belt. Without its presence, our bodies cannot properly produce DHEA, progesterone, estrogen, testosterone, and hydrocortisone. Pregnenolone, which is also produced in the brain, also affects many neurotransmitters.

Like all other hormones, pregnenolone declines with age. Many doctors use pregnenolone to treat memory problems, depression, and fatigue, and it can be helpful with autoimmune conditions.

As with all hormones, clinical doses go a long way in our ability to function and be well. At fifty, we shouldn't be producing anything near what we did at twenty of *any* hormone. A dose of ten to twenty-five milligrams per day of pregnenolone is all that is necessary.

NATURAL ESTROGEN

Natural estrogen is such a controversial issue. I will do my best to try to explain why that is the case and why most, but not all, doctors are defensive about it and against it.

A woman produces three types of estrogen: 80 percent estriol, 10 percent estrone, and 10 percent estradiol. When a woman begins menopause, wouldn't it be common sense to make sure that these three estrogens continue to be replaced in her body in the same percentage? One with common sense would think so.

Premarin, which is the most common synthetic estrogen, comes from a pregnant mare and consists of mostly estrone. Estrace, which is another popular synthetic drug, consists of all estradiol. Premarin and Estrace do not contain all three of the above-mentioned estrogen types. So where are the 80 percent estriol, 10 percent estrone, and 10 percent estradiol in my body if I am given either Premarin or Estrace? I guess a pregnant mare and I don't have much in common after all.

Estradiol is the greatest stimulator of breast tissue. According to the Journal of the American Medical Association, January 26, 2000, there is a forty percent risk increase of breast cancer and endometrial hyperplasia while on their synthetic estrogen therapies. They were being overstimulated with the wrong estrogen(s). None of these synthetic prescriptions contain estriol. Estriol is usually the only form of estrogen needed after menopause. After all, we are not in the baby-making business anymore, are we? Our biggest concern now becomes strong bones and heart health. Estriol will also keep your skin and other tissue youthful.

When choosing a doctor to get you through menopause (before, during, and after), find one who knows the correct blood work and saliva tests to perform on you. This will ensure that your compounded prescription is geared toward you getting the estrogen(s), as well as other hormones, you need for *your* body now. Remember, girls, all estrogen is not created equal!

When taking estrogen, you must take *natural* progesterone. If not, you will be estrogen dominant. If there is not enough progesterone in your body, estrogen cannot do its job. They work together as partners.

NATURAL PROGESTERONE

Wow! Where do I begin to talk about this amazing hormone? For those of us who have been pregnant, we remember that deep, wonderful sleep the first trimester. The loss of this hormone is one reason why women going through menopause are sleep deprived.

Women produce this hormone in both the ovaries and in small amounts in the adrenals. Besides being necessary for the survival of the fetus, it can serve on many other levels.

It can stimulate cells for bone building, therefore assisting with osteoporosis. It can also normalize blood sugar and assist thyroid function. Many experienced doctors will prescribe natural progesterone to treat endometriosis, PMS, depression, and fibrocystic breast and uterine disease. It can also assist with water retention and libido. I have read about many cases of postpartum depression resulting from the drastic drop in progesterone after birth.

Natural progesterone is made from plant products and has the same chemical structure our body makes. Provera, which is synthetic, has been chemically altered. Because of this alteration, the human body has no receptors to absorb synthetic progesterone. Pharmaceutical companies cannot patent a natural substance, as the law currently states. You do not have to be going through menopause to have hormone imbalances. How many thirty-year-old women do you know who have any of the symptoms above?

MELATONIN

Melatonin is a hormone secreted from the pineal gland, located in the brain. Tryptophan, which is an amino acid, is a precursor to serotonin. Serotonin then converts into melatonin. Serotonin is a neurotransmitter associated with depression.

In addition to improving sleep, melatonin is a strong antioxidant good for the immune system. As we age, melatonin, DHEA, and human growth hormone decline.

The pineal gland controls our twenty-four-hour clock known as our circadian rhythm. In addition to aging, stress and anxiety contribute to this imbalance. Overproduction of hydrocortisone will inhibit secretion of melatonin. Treating the adrenals in addition to melatonin is equally important.

Clinical dosages are what we need. Usually a dose of only one-half milligram to a maximum of three milligrams is sufficient. It is just enough to assist our bodies to secrete melatonin on its own again.

When going through stressful times, I always take five hundred milligrams of magnesium with my melatonin and one-quarter to one-half cup of dark cherry juice before bedtime. Magnesium will block hydrocortisone and allow the melatonin to work. They work together to achieve sleep. Cherry juice stops any inflammation present in the tissues of the body. If you experience drowsiness the next day, cut down your milligrams of melatonin.

Chapter Four
Genetic Nutrition

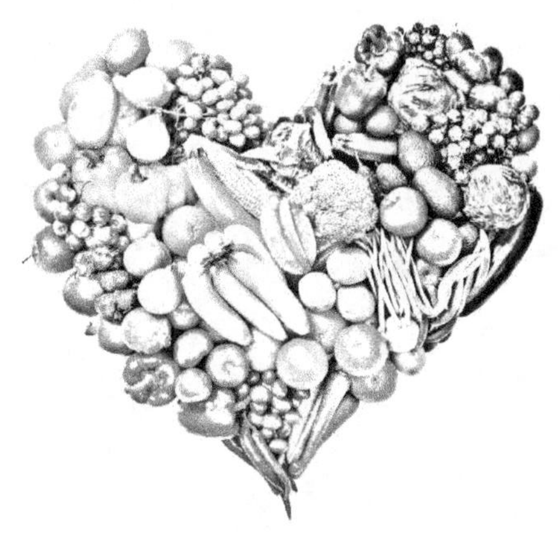

4

Genetic Nutrition

Let food be thy medicine and medicine be thy food.

—Hippocrates

I considered leaving this chapter blank. If I wrote about every food the media has an issue with, there would be nothing nutritious for us to eat—except bottled water. I decided to take it from a genetic standpoint. We are all unique, as our creator intended. Hopefully this will help everyone to understand why there is so much controversy about what to eat and which diet to follow.

APOLIPOPROTEIN E (APO E)

Did you ever wonder why when your friends go on a new eating plan, they lose weight, feel great, and have lots of energy and why when you follow the same plan, the outcome is not the same? I'm convinced that if every one of us was tested for this genotype, there would be no question what we, as individuals, need to eat not just for weight control but also for heart disease and inflammation present in the body.

Simply put, the Apo E gene regulates the way your body transports cholesterol and fats. There are three variants of this gene: E2, E3, and E4. A human cell has two copies of each gene. Therefore, it creates six genotypes. Everyone inherits two copies of this gene, one from each parent. The six are E2/E2, E3/E3, E4/E4, E2/E3, E2/E4, and E3/E4.

I will break this down as easily as possible. I'm not a genetic doctor, as I'm sure most reading this are not! Before I go any further, I must stress how important cholesterol is to our body. It is important for our nervous system, cell membranes, hormone function, and vitamin-D assimilation. As you will read below, there is more to good health than just a cholesterol panel your doctor orders up for you.

According to Pamela McDonald, integrative medicine fellow and author of *The Apo E Gene Diet: A Breakthrough in Changing Cholesterol, Weight, Heart, and Alzheimer's Using the Body's Own Genes*, 80 percent of people who develop coronary artery disease have the same total cholesterol level as those who did not develop the disease. That's because there are twelve different subtypes of cholesterol particles contained in the two major LDL and HDL groups. And yes, these tests are available and affordable.

An E2 carrier has the lowest risk of coronary heart disease due to low LDL cholesterol. E3 carriers make up approximately 60 percent of the population and have a normal level of cholesterol. E4 carriers have high LDL, which makes them more susceptible to coronary heart disease, atherosclerosis, and sadly Alzheimer's disease.

The hope would be that you are a combination-gene type, as being an E2/E2 or an E4/E4 would restrict a wider variety of food types. E2 carriers do much better on a higher fat and very low carb and sugar diet. (And yes—sorry to say, friends—no alcohol. No matter what Apo E you are, it doesn't give you a ticket to eat processed food and sugar and to drink excessive alcohol.) Such carriers should eat lots of vegetables, nuts, olives, olive oil, coconut, coconut oil, sweet potatoes, some legumes, eggs, animal protein, and some fruit. The diet should be about 30 to 35 percent fat.

What do you think would happen if an E2 didn't eat this way? Since cholesterol may not be the issue, I can almost assure you that type 2 diabetes and/or pancreas issues can result from poor eating habits. All of this can lead to coronary plaque and heart disease eventually.

Take me for example. I am an E2/E3. Ninety percent of the time, I eat as listed above (E2). The E3 in me allows me to have a few carbs a week other than sweet potatoes. I do not drink. I feel horrible when I do so even occasionally. There is no coronary heart disease on either side of my family. However, my maternal grandfather became diabetic at fifty and died at sixty-five of pancreatic cancer. My paternal grandfather also died of pancreatic cancer. And my father currently has a less aggressive form of pancreatic cancer, which starts in the hormone-producing cells of the pancreas. Both sides have Italian decent, and none of them were overweight. However, I guess the bread and pasta on a daily basis was a bad idea for them, and I'm sure they are bad for me too!

Environment, stress management, and proper exercise may have lessened their risk for the above diseases. A body in a constant state of stress can still have disease no matter what the person eats. Look around your world. Are the aesthetics in your home and work calming? Do you surround yourself with people who are pleasant, aware, and like-minded? What are your spiritual and religious beliefs? Are you meditating? Our thoughts control our total body chemistry.

It is interesting that before genetic blood work, all clinical nutritionists who have either tested my muscle or taken a hair analysis from me have told me to eat this way for the past thirty years. At the present time, I have no issues with cholesterol or diabetes.

E4s should be eating low fat, only about 20 percent of the diet per day. Protein should come from mostly plant sources, and they should have complex carbohydrates high in fiber but no refined carbohydrates (for any of us). There should be lots of vegetables and fruits for these E4 carriers. If you are a E3/E4 or an E2/E4, you can add fish to your protein sources. If you are an E4 carrier, eat a high fat diet; chances are that your LDL cholesterol can cause inflammation in the blood vessels, including those in the brain, which is the connection to Alzheimer's.

Taking all the right precautions may not guarantee you will not get any of the above-listed diseases, but postponing *any* disease is a victory!

METHYLENETETRAHYDROFOLATE REDUCTASE (MTHFR MUTATION)

It's hard enough to pronounce much less explain. Before I go any further, it is important to know the function of B vitamins. They help convert our food into fuel so that we have sufficient energy. B vitamins are essential for our hair, skin, and nails, and they are very critical to our liver and nervous system. They are water-soluble, so we need to be sure that we are getting more than enough, especially at highly stressful times.

The MTHFR gene is an enzyme that properly helps make folate (B9) usable in the body. Usable folate in the body is called methylfolate. This breakdown process is called methylation. If there is not enough methylfolate, your body will not be able to convert homocysteine into methionine. Methionine is an amino acid that helps the body process and eliminate fat. This amino acid contains sulfur, which helps produce a very important natural antioxidant in our body called glutathione (GSH). If levels of homocysteine are too high, the person can be at risk for cardiovascular issues, such as heart attack, stroke, neuropathy, and blood clots. Put simply if a person tests positive for this genetic mutation, then converting folate into a usable form is not possible.

In addition to the above health risks, methylfolate is critical for neurotransmitter and DNA production, detoxification, and immune function. Neurotransmitter imbalance can highly affect mood, sleep, anxiety, depression, motivation, and overall energy. Other symptoms are migraines, memory loss, dementia, Alzheimer's, and many other neurological or psychological issues, depending on how you manifest the imbalance, I suppose.

As mentioned above, GSH is an antioxidant also produced from methylfolate. GSH prevents damage to our cells and helps to fight the free radicals and to detoxify heavy metals from our body. Without sufficient detoxification and enough antioxidants, DNA damage is at risk. How does our immune system fight cancer and other diseases?

Folic acid is a synthetic form of folate. You know, it's what all the doctors tell you to take when you are pregnant to prevent spina bifida. Taking synthetic folic acid either in food or supplements is even worse—whether you have this mutation or not. (And it is in everything. Read your labels well.) If you are a nonmethylator, it's just building up in your organs and tissue. Folate is present in raw, green leafy vegetables. This is much better than folic acid, but help will still be needed to receive all the benefits above.

So how do we shut off this mutation? First of all, take 5-MTHF supplement, which is methylfolate. I also take a probiotic, fermented B complex, which bypasses this mutation and enters right into my liver, for immediate energy, adrenal-gland support, and immune-system and mood balance. In addition to 5-MTHF, you can take a supplement known as calcium D-glucarate. Calcium D-glucarate assists the liver in a process known as glucuronidation. Glucuronidation is a specific detoxification system that has been shown to help excrete lipid-soluble toxins and steroid hormones out of the body. I believe it would be wise to take this supplement with this mutation.

Second, *detoxify*! Do everything you can to stimulate the lymphatic system. Studies have shown that exercising can slow down Alzheimer's. Why? Because sweating is a form of detoxification. Everyone should drink lots of filtered water in glass, not plastic, and avoid using microwave ovens as much as possible. You are trying not to ingest chemicals from plastic and to keep as much nutrition in your food as possible. If you must occasionally use a microwave, *do not* heat in plastic. Try to consume vegetables and fruits, as they are high in water content.

Massages and jumping on a minitrampoline will stimulate lymph flow. You should have contact with no perfumes or harsh chemicals, and sorry—once again—you should not drink alcohol. And as I will explain in the "Alternative Remedies" chapter, you should use castor-oil packs and colonics. And as for all good health, quality sleep, if possible. Good sleep could be an issue with this mutation. All the above is critical for me especially. I have tested positive for this mutation. Let's have a look at my environment. I teach movement to people all day, and I am exposed to their detoxifying sweat. Then I give them a massage. So first I breathe it in, and then I touch it. Yikes. Not good.

Ladies, this paragraph is for all of you who complain about getting your monthly menstrual cycle. That is one of nature's greatest detoxifications. I believe the lack of this monthly detoxification to be one reason why many women gain weight after menopause. Your body just lost one pathway to get rid of a whole lot of toxins. And if you have this mutation, it just got even harder. Please do not complain about that once-a-month visit. Because within a year after menopause, it is a race against time on the aging train, both with how you look and how you feel.

Other genetic factors matter also. This explains many things about my body, such as how horrible I feel when I drink alcohol. Because if you remember, my Apo E is a 2/3, which means no alcohol, and methylation is a challenge for me. That's a double whammy for me. But thank goodness, I do not have a four in my Apo E genotype. If so, I would be *very* concerned about dementia, Alzheimer's, and other debilitating neurological disorders. Just because you are taking proper supplementation and living life clean, it doesn't give you a ticket to do whatever you want. Occasional cheats are OK, but not daily for sure. After all, we do need to allow ourselves to be human and enjoy life. Once again, it's not only genes that matter but also the way that you nurture your emotional and spiritual self.

VITAMIN D

Are we allergic to food, or are we increasingly allergic to what has been done to it?

—Robyn O'Brien

All of a sudden over the past couple years, the medical world has jumped on this one. It's funny how most doctors tell us we don't need to take vitamins; we just have to eat well. That would be great if our soil was filled with nutrients like it used to be and our vegetables came from yard to table within a day, if our dairy was unpasteurized and our grains processed properly. And that is why they now give prescriptions for vitamin D. I guess that's all the medical world thinks we need. It is a good start but certainly not the complete answer.

Vitamin-D deficiencies can lead to calcium, iron, magnesium, phosphate, and zinc deficiencies, all of which can lead to skeletal disease, autoimmune disease, metabolic issues, cancer, all sorts of infections, and even cognitive disorders.

Vitamin D is a fat-soluble vitamin received from the sun and in foods. D2 is in plant-based foods, and D3 is in foods such as egg yolks, fatty fish, liver, and cod-liver oil. That is why the Norwegians eat so much of these foods in their diet, since they have long winters with no sun. Our government also thought it was healthier for us all to eat vegetable oils instead of animal shortening. Now suddenly, we are all vitamin-D deficient. Hmm. I guess that canola oil isn't working!

D3 can be made internally when the body is exposed to the sun. Let us think about this. We are always covered in sunscreen, which keeps our bodies from absorbing ultraviolet rays. Fifteen minutes of sun a day is all it takes to get sufficient amounts of vitamin D. Dermal synthesis of vitamin D from cholesterol can only happen with sun exposure. We store vitamin D on the dermal layer of skin, so if you are constantly soaping up and putting lotion on your skin, you are washing it away.

"Now she doesn't want me to use soap?" you might be asking. I think that maybe you should only soap your extremities every other day. I use sunscreen only when I know I will be in the sun for a long period of time. If you use body lotion, use shea butter. It has some vitamin D in it, and it is a natural sunscreen. Find a good vitamin-D supplement. I would avoid prescription-based vitamin D. Why? You can't patent a natural substance. In order to make it available through a pharmacy, there has to be something else in it. I know the supplement vitamin D will be better absorbed as natural as possible.

I eat an entire egg. The media has given God's most perfect food a bad reputation. The color alone tells you the amount of nutrients in the yolk, such as lutein and zeaxanthin, which are great for your eyes. There are also vitamins A, D, E, and K; calcium; phosphorus; zinc; selenium; iron; choline; magnesium; folate; and vitamins B5, B12, and B2—to name a few!

The egg has a bit of every nutrient we need. To get the most nutritional value out of eggs (as any food), eat as close to raw as possible, either soft-boiled or poached minimally.

It is not cholesterol that is bad for us. It is the *oxidation* of cholesterol that leads to plaque in the arteries. And that, my friends, is an overcooked scrambled or hard-boiled egg. The liver produces cholesterol daily to feed our organs. If we eat eggs, our liver just may not have to produce so much to keep it all going. I had a clinical nutritionist tell me years ago that people with an allergy to eggs are most likely to be allergic to the whites. What does that tell you?

There is more to being healthy than just keeping your weight down by eating egg whites. Besides do you really think America got high cholesterol and became overweight eating eggs? I doubt it. I am currently fifty-four, and I have twenty-twenty vision. I am going to keep eating my soft-boiled and poached eggs.

Also, the best and most highly absorbed calcium available to us is eggshells. We throw them away and buy expensive calcium supplements that none of us can absorb. After cracking open a raw egg, dry the shells out for a day or more, if you want to collect them for a while. Steam them on top of the stove for sterilization, let them dry, and grind them up in the blender, Vitamix, or coffee grinder to a fine powder. You can fill gelatin caps and have your own supplements, or you can store the powder in a glass jar and put a teaspoon a day in your food with smoothies, sweet potatoes, and so on. When my dogs have dietary needs, I make their food. I always put powdered egg shells in it for calcium.

Most of us usually need more vitamin D than the FDA's daily recommendations. Start out with two thousand units per day, and see how you feel. Most times, we need far more than two thousand units per day. You may adjust accordingly.

APPLE-CIDER VINEGAR

There are so many reasons to use apple-cider vinegar in your daily routine. When apple juice is fermented and left raw, unfiltered, and unpasteurized, the benefits are additional enzymes, trace minerals, probiotics, and pectin. The highest quality is cloudy with stringy particles floating in it. People spend so much money on digestive enzyme supplements. All you need is one tablespoon of apple-cider vinegar to one cup of water before meals. Vinegar will cleanse and detoxify your digestive system, gallbladder, and liver.

Studies have shown that regular use of apple-cider vinegar at meals can block a surge in blood-glucose levels. This happens no matter what you eat. That is why I am not a big fan of the multiple-meals-a-day theory. However, drinking apple-cider vinegar doesn't give you a free pass to eat anything you want either. Constant spikes in glucose levels can lead to not only diabetes but also to high cholesterol and cardiovascular disease.

Drinking apple-cider vinegar will help the body stay alkaline so your immune system can fight off illness much more efficiently.

I also put apple-cider vinegar in my bath water, especially when I feel as though my body may be trying to fight off a cold or virus. I use three cups to a full tub. I assure that you will not smell like a big salad. The addition of three cups of vinegar is not much to a tub of water.

I also put it in my dogs' water. The vinegar will repel fleas and mosquitoes very effectively, and it will assist in the dogs' digestive health also. Insects do not like an alkaline body—yours or theirs!

And finally, I use it in my yard. It will keep the mold off your plants and lawn. In larger concentration levels, it is a great weed killer. Apple-cider vinegar is a natural way to cut down chemicals from hurting you, your pets, and all God's natural habitat.

Chapter Five
Alternative Remedies

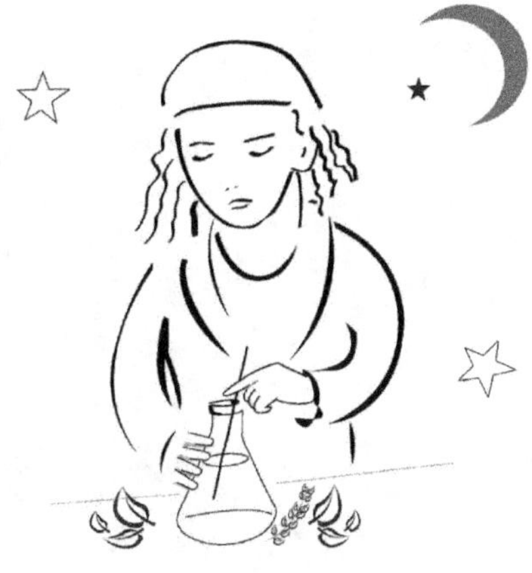

5

Alternative Remedies

With the past, I have nothing to do; nor with the future. I live now.

—Ralph Waldo Emerson

The natural healing force within each of us is the greatest force in getting well.

—Hippocrates

There are so many wonderful remedies available for healing. Maybe you have heard of the options I have listed below. I hope this can clarify some unanswered questions you may have about them. If it resonates with you, that usually means you would benefit from it. If it doesn't now, it may someday. As with anyone whom you are entrusting your health and wellness with, be sure to seek out certified and licensed practitioners.

YOUR BODY DOESN'T LIE

Behavioral kinesiology is based on the book written by John Diamond, MD, *Your Body Doesn't Lie: Unlock the Power of Your Natural Energy!* A philosophy as well as an integrated science, behavioral kinesiology spans all the healing arts. It has been incorporated into many diverse areas of psychosomatic medicine, allergy, acupuncture, psychiatry, nutrition, dentistry, osteopathy, and sports training as well as veterinarian use.

During testing, you may use the deltoid muscle or the finger. A person being tested will hold one arm out straight as another person pushes down on the arm while asking a very specific question, such as, "Am I allergic to peanuts?" If the arm of the person being tested stays firm and strong, the answer is yes. If the muscle weakens and the arm goes down, the answer is no. As mentioned above, this test can also be done while pressing the thumb and the third finger together firmly while other person applies pressure outward. If the fingers stay strongly in contact with each other, the answer is yes. If they weaken and come apart, the answer is no. The person being tested can hold the food or supplement against their stomach for an accurate result. If it is a supplement, you can get very specific with questions, including those about specific brands and dosage, frequency, and duration.

Muscle testing is the way I determine what to eat, which remedies to use, and how much to use. The most important thing to remember is always treat *in the moment*. The body is always changing. What you needed yesterday may not be what you need today. I use this type of testing on myself, my family, my animals, and my clients.

There are no two of us alike. This is why there are so many different opinions on diet and nutrition. Eat dairy; don't eat dairy. Should I eat wheat or not? Should I be a vegetarian? Do I need this remedy? If so, how much, for how long, and how frequently?

Many clinical nutritionists use—along with hair analysis—saliva testing and now the proof of science from all the various blood labs.

Think it's a scam? I have blown some people's minds away with muscle testing. Both with humans and animals. Not to mention the amazing results from muscle testing. It has never failed me. Remember, your body's own innate wisdom knows what it needs. We are all connected to God and spirit, and that is where truth prevails.

MEDITATION

We come for the healing of the soul, the mind, and the heart, knowing that all else will follow as the healing of the body.

—Archangel Raphael

Meditation is a form of relaxation through breath. The autonomic nervous system (ANS) controls this vital function. Your breath is the only part of the ANS that is consciously controllable. Doesn't something we do so many times a day deserve more awareness and attention than most of us currently give it?

When the mind creates a better sense of well-being, stress, anxiety, digestion, and lowered blood pressure are all results of a healthier physical, mental, and emotional body. Therefore, we are allowing our spirit to achieve all we came here to do. There is no better way to heal the body and receive guidance than meditation. It is available at our disposal at no cost. Yet it is the most difficult practice for most people.

I believe the reason is that we are not willing to create the time each day to quiet our analytical minds because we think of meditation as not being productive. Not performing meditation is why our breath becomes shallow and we have pain everywhere. Your breath and lungs are about how you take in life. Do you take in life fully with love or shallow with fear?

I know there are many people who think it is so "new age" to meditate. I ask, "If all you do is pray all the time, how do you suppose you are going to receive your messages from God and spirit with all the constant mental chatter?" We must listen from our hearts, not our minds. One of my favorite things to do is go to church before services begin and just sit quietly and receive my messages. The rosary (and other types of prayer beads) is also a form of meditation. It helps create a calming inner awareness of faith, as do many religious repetitive rituals. What does faith mean to you? For me, it is trusting what is unseen.

Taking fifteen minutes a day to meditate can make you accomplish much more in your day with a clearer mind and a calmer spirit. And all of that, my friends, leads to a healthy body.

HEAL YOUR BODY

Louise Hay is an author who has dedicated her writings toward helping people understand the mental causes for our physical illnesses and the metaphysical ways to overcome them.

What an amazing woman. Sexually abused as a child, she later was diagnosed with vaginal cancer. When practicing positive affirmations in meditation, she totally released all cancer. She needed no surgery and has been cancer-free for many years. Wow! Imagine the awe the doctors had.

This quick reference guide lists the physical issue or "dis-ease" we are experiencing, followed by the mental thought patterns that form our experience, and lastly ways to replace these old thought patterns with wonderful new healing affirmations.

Whenever I am experiencing issues with my body, I look up the issue in her book and make it a point to repeat the associated affirmations throughout the day. It is so interesting to discover that most of these patterns are rooted in criticism, anger, resentment, and guilt. It is a wonderful discovery about what has manifested in our subconscious.

When the need to continue smoking, having anxiety, and so on is gone, the outer effect must die. As she states, "If you kill the root, the plant will die."

The power of forgiveness *is* an amazing thing.

COLONICS

All disease begins in the gut.

—Hippocrates

I know what you are thinking: I can't believe she's going there. Well, I am! The first colonic dates back in Egyptian history as early as 1500 BC.

ACUPUNCTURE

Acupuncture originated in China more than two thousand five hundred years ago. Western medicine is finally coming around to realizing the many benefits of this remedy. In traditional Chinese medicine, acupuncture works with what are called meridians (lines of energy that flow throughout the body, sometimes referred to as "chi"). When this energy becomes imbalanced, dis-ease begins.

According to Andrew Weil, MD, research published in the May 30, 2010, edition of *Nature Neuroscience*, was the proof that Western medicine was looking for regarding the benefits of acupuncture. Apparently, there is an amino acid, adenosine, that is released through the skin after any injury, and this amino acid naturally eases pain. According to Dr. Weil, the needles entering the skin will create a subtle injury to produce this effect. This is why so many people experience a relief from pain immediately following a session.

I'll buy that. However, I believe the Eastern concept more. I have been doing acupuncture for about twenty-five years. My first visit was for acne. I went twice a week. After the first month, I never had an issue again. Since then I have received acupuncture on a regular basis. I find acupuncture to be good for many emotional, digestive, and neurological issues, such as anxiety, depression, insomnia, endocrine imbalances, headaches, and respiratory problems. The list goes on and on. Acupuncture is cumulative. Treat the issue consistently, and then you can back off with a maintenance program for overall energy balance. Sometimes there will be an herbal remedy recommended to go along with treatments.

The acupuncturist will give you a thorough screening on your first session. This screening includes questioning you about medications and diet, checking your pulse, and examining your tongue. These will tell the acupuncturist where your imbalances are and how to begin appropriate treatment. I'll leave you with this. My acupuncturist was the first person to tell me I was two weeks pregnant—and I was. My son is now ten years old!

HOMEOPATHY

Samuel Hahnemann was born in Germany in 1755. Despite his family's inability to pay for education, his great intellect was noticed by many teachers, and he was admitted to college and later the University of Leipzig to study medicine. While working on a translation project, he came across a particular tree bark known as cinchona from South America used to treat malaria-induced fever. When he ingested this bark, he realized that it caused all the same symptoms as malaria.

Hahnemann's discovery of homeopathy is based on the belief that like cures like. For example, whatever causes illness in a healthy person can cure the patient. Hahnemann also believed that our mental, emotional, and spiritual belief systems can contribute to habitual patterns of behavior, which can cause disease to not fully heal.

Most medical doctors roll their eyes at this form of treatment. My question to them would be, "Isn't that similar to how vaccinations work?" Shoot a bit of the germ in our body so that we build immunity to it. Why is that theory recognized for vaccines and nothing else? Heaven forbid we treat anything in the medical world past the physical body. Why not treat it all? With homeopathy, we are treating so many other issues, possibly before they turn into something worse.

My son hates taking medicine of any kind. Outside of the common cold, he has never been sick. If I see the signs, I immediately get him started on a homeopathic remedy. Fortunately, he hates taking medicine more than having a runny nose. Therefore, he doesn't seem to be bothered at all by discomfort. He will take the homeopathic remedy but will fight me tooth and nail about taking anything else.

When he was nine years old, the doctor lanced a cyst that had formed on his body and prescribed antibiotics. I was exhausted bartering with him every day to get that medicine down his throat. But guess what. I believed he needed to take it. However, I don't think we should take antibiotics for every little ailment. If we do, we don't respond to them when needed, and our immune system weakens overall.

Antibiotics kill all the great flora in our digestive system, as I discuss in my chapter on the organs. I believe that is why my son is rarely ill. So many illnesses will run their course in a few days to a week if we are patient enough to sit with them. In addition to treating myself and my family, I also use homeopathy on my animals. I always get a positive response. I have my kit of one hundred remedies in my medicine cabinet. When I travel, it goes along, too. Some of the issues I treat are bee stings, bug bites, and upset stomach, to name a few.

I believe we *all* need to have respect for the many avenues of treatment that are available to us and to know that there is a correct time and place for choosing the appropriate prescription.

CRYOTHERAPY

Whole-body cryotherapy is becoming increasingly popular in many populations not just with competitive athletes. Very low temperatures are known to have anti-inflammatory and antioxidant effects on the body. By treating inflammation, the benefits can be endless. Possible benefits include reduced arthritis and joint pain, quicker surgical recovery, more efficient metabolism, better overall blood circulation, and better lymphatic system drainage, which will help eliminate toxins from the body. Until recently, there had been much controversy on whether it has legitimate results.

In 2016, at the congress of the International Psychogeriatric Association, Dr. Joanna Rymaszewska, MD, PhD, of Wroclaw Medical University in Poland said that whole-body cryotherapy has been known to ease depression, help prevent dementia, and improve symptoms in patients with mild cognitive impairment. Remembering back to my first treatment, I became so relaxed immediately after. It was as if I was shot with a tranquilizer. It felt like a complete reset of my nervous system. No pain or tension anywhere—followed by a great night sleep. My first three treatments were a repeat. I now leave feeling highly energized. I did notice an increase in my appetite within the first month and a two-pound weight loss. I currently visit the tank once a week.

You can read endless opinions on cryotherapy. If an ice pack can bring blood circulation to an injured area, why can't the same benefit help with full-body circulation and healing? Seems logical to me. It's interesting though that most skeptics have never experienced it. I try, as with most treatments, to pay attention to how I feel and not focus entirely on what I read. And as with any wellness remedy, you must be consistent for a while before drawing any conclusions.

CASTOR-OIL PACKS (PALMA CHRISTI)

It is easy to get a thousand prescriptions but hard to get one single remedy.

—CHINESE PROVERB

Edgar Cayce was an American Christian known as "the sleeping prophet." He was given a beautiful gift from God to serve humanity. From a self-induced trance, he was able to answer questions about health and healing in individuals who sought him out for help. Every reading was documented and filed in his library in Virginia Beach, Virginia, known as the Association of Research and Enlightenment (ARE). It is the second largest library in the world, next to the Vatican. And I have been there. What an unbelievable place of healing. I have read many of his case histories, as I am a member of the ARE and have access to the histories online. One amazing story after another about everyone's unique journey for answers regarding health and spirit. No two are alike, as expected.

Castor-oil packs were very common in folk medicine. Cayce used this form of therapy for many illnesses: tumors, constipation, adhesions, cataracts, digestion issues, gallstones, epilepsy, migraines, lymphadenitis, and toxemia—to name a few. All healing starts by stimulating the lymphatic system and boosting the immune system, which is what is happening with these packs.

A flannel pack is saturated with cold-pressed castor oil and then applied to the area of treatment. It is followed by plastic wrap, towel, heating pad, and another towel to hold the heat into the body. After removing the flannel pack, you sponge off the oil with warm water and baking soda. Frequency and length of time vary with each person. Most times a small dose of olive oil is to be taken after treatment. This is necessary to flush the intestines, continue lymphatic drainage, and detoxify the liver. (He believed in colonics also.)

Once again, we see the importance of cleaning out the organs and intestines. These packs are so comforting, and yes, they *do* work. The healing property is a fatty acid known as ricinoleic acid. The plant was known as the palma Christi, because the leaves were said to resemble the hand of Christ.

I strongly suggest you read more about Cayce and the many health issues he assisted in healing. My favorite book is *The Edgar Cayce Handbook for Health Through Drugless Therapy*. There are countless books written about him and his wonderful gifts and talents. You can become a member of the ARE and have access to his entire library online—every reading he did. The ARE can also guide you to doctors and nurses who are familiar with administering his treatments.

BACH FLOWER ESSENCES

We can judge our health by our happiness.

—EDWARD BACH

The earth laughs in flowers.

—RALPH WALDO EMERSON

Edward Bach was a British medical doctor, pathologist, bacteriologist, and homeopath in the 1930s. He developed the thirty-eight flower-essence remedies known as Bach flower remedies. He believed that diseases result from imbalances or negativity at the soul level. He studied the link between emotional states of his patients and disease, and he realized that flowers had healing properties that could be very beneficial.

Flower essences are created by placing a flower or part of a plant in water, placing it in sunlight, and allowing the water to take on the vibrational energies of that particular plant. They are very gentle. They cannot cause any harm even while the person using them is on medications. There are no side effects or risks of overdosing. If the incorrect blend is chosen, there will be no harm.

The best remedy is a custom blend, one that is made specifically for you. However, if you are going through a difficult time with something now, that doesn't mean that same custom remedy will work for you next year. Our mental, spiritual, physical, and emotional bodies are always changing and evolving. I have custom-blended Bach remedies for myself, my son, my clients, and—yes—even my pets.

One remedy I use very frequently for panic, anxiety, or any kind of stress relief is Rescue Remedy, Bach's most popular remedy. It is always mixed up in the fridge for emergency use. I give this to my dogs before they go to the vet or during a thunderstorm. I give it to my son if he is hurt and can't calm down. I used it daily while remodeling my house. It can be taken orally or rubbed on ears or paws.

Bach remedies need to be diluted, add four drops into a glass, one-ounce (thirty-milliliter) dropper bottle. Add water not quite to the top so that you leave room for dropper. Shake well, and store in fridge for up to six weeks. If you want to carry it with you without refrigeration, then add one dropperful of apple-cider vinegar to bottle to preserve the blend. Before taking, shake well. Only two to four drops are needed. It should be taken usually two to three times daily. Be your own best judge of the frequency, depending on the severity of the situation. Be sure not to let dropper touch the mouth or anything, as it will contaminate the rest of your blend.

AROMATHERAPY: MEDICINE FROM THE EARTH

Nature always wears the color of the spirit.

—Ralph Waldo Emerson

Essential oils are one of the greatest medicinal resources for healing from our earth. Essential oils are extracted from flowers, herbs, bark, seeds, roots, leaves, and fruits. Aromatherapy has been used for centuries all over the world, dating back to Egypt over five thousand years ago. In modern times, we have forgotten the power that comes from our earth. For example, oregano is twenty-six times more powerful an antiseptic than phenol, which is found in most cleaning products.

These oils can be inhaled from the bottle or a diffuser or diluted in a carrier like oil, lotion, or water and applied to the skin. They can affect people or animals physically, mentally, emotionally, and spiritually.

When the olfactory gland senses smell, endorphins (which relieve pain), serotonin (which is calming), and noradrenaline (which stimulates rejuvenation) release. This gland is also responsible for stimulating the part of your brain where memories and emotions are stored. After the brain processes, the molecules enter the bloodstream and travel throughout the body. This results in full-body healing.

Essential oils are used in many products, such as soaps, lotions, candles, shampoos, bath salts, room mists, cleaners, and mouthwash.

Caution needs to be taken by everyone when using essential oils. Caution should especially be taken with children and animals and during pregnancy. It is always wise to seek advice from a certified aromatherapist if there is something specific you are treating and if you are uncertain about safety.

In Europe, oils are routinely taken internally, but there is a large community of trained allopathic and naturopathic doctors who can safely prescribe. It is not recommended to take them orally. Essential oils are so easily absorbed into the circulatory system that there is no reason to ingest them.

If I had to choose oils for the average home to have in the medicine cabinet, I would choose lavender, tea tree, chamomile, peppermint, eucalyptus, geranium, thyme, rosemary, and lemon.

Lavender: This oil is capable of many treatments. Every home should have this, if no other. It is great with burns, wounds, insomnia, and respiratory conditions. It is a natural antibiotic, antiseptic, sedative, and detoxifier. Use of lavender can contribute to quick cell regeneration of wounds. Take caution with low blood pressure and early pregnancy, since most women's blood pressure drops at this time.

Tea Tree: This is antiviral, antifungal, and antibacterial. The antiseptic properties of this oil are one hundred times more than those of carbolic acid, but it is nontoxic to humans. It can be used to treat acne, wounds, and toothaches, and it can be used in mouthwashes and for any type of fungus, such as athlete's foot.

Chamomile: There are both German and Roman chamomile. These are both excellent for the nervous system and insomnia. Chamomile is an antibacterial disinfectant, and it is good for inflammation, such as arthritis. It is great for children to help them calm down when ill. Use either a couple of drops in a bath or a diffuser in the bedroom.

Eucalyptus: This is best known for its use in treatment against bronchial issues such as coughing and colds. This is also anti-inflammatory, antibacterial, antibiotic, analgesic, antiviral, deodorizing, and diuretic. Eucalyptus is a great insect repellent.

Geranium: This is infused not from the flower geranium but from the *Pelargonium* lemon plant. It is awesome for skin care, menopause, blood disorders, and diabetes, and geranium is a great sedative for the nerves.

Rosemary: This oil is used for all muscular conditions, such as arthritis, fatigue, headaches, diabetes, flu, memory loss, and depression. It is great in beauty treatments for hair, acne, and cellulite.

Make your own first-aid spray with any of these. Use eight drops of essential oil to four ounces of water. Shake well. If you want to blend any of these oils, blend in a dropper bottle. Shake well, and then add eights drops of the blend to water or your carrier of choice.

I have put together many great stress blends. I will give you one of my favorite blends. Take a dropper bottle, and mix fifty drops of orange, thirty drops of lavender, and fifteen drops of ylang ylang. Shake well, and add eight to ten drops to four ounces of water or carrier oil, such as grapeseed, almond, or jojoba oil. This blend is quite euphoric.

CRANIOSACRAL THERAPY (CST)

This therapy was developed by osteopath John Upledger. During a surgery, he noticed rhythmic movement of the craniosacral system that led him to believe that he could manipulate the synarthrodial (a type of joint that permits little or no movement) joints of the cranium and create movement in the brain and spinal cord with little pressure on specific points of the body. There is much controversy in the medical world challenging Upledger's belief that the bones of the skull can shift. The craniosacral system consists of the membranes and cerebrospinal fluid that surround and protect the brain and spinal cord. It extends from the bones of the skull, face, and mouth, which make up the cranium, down to the sacrum or tailbone.

CST can help treat imbalances in the brain and spinal cord, which can lead to any number of sensory, motor, or neurological disabilities. These problems can include chronic pain, eye difficulties, scoliosis, motor-coordination impairments, learning disabilities, and many other health challenges.

I have been a craniosacral therapist since 1999. I have had many clients come to me for treatment. They mostly come for headaches and TMJ issues. All are very surprised at what they feel. As a therapist giving this treatment, I can feel movement in my hands from the client's body. When I personally receive CST, it starts out with a pulsating feeling, and then it's as if my body is floating gently on a raft. The ongoing response is, "I feel something moving." Feedback has always been positive after treatment. This therapy is very gentle and quite relaxing to receive.

REIKI

> *Just as a candle cannot burn without fire, men cannot live without a spiritual life.*
>
> —BUDDHA

Reiki is a Japanese word that means "universal life energy." We are all born with it.

Reiki was brought to us before World War II by a man named Mikao Usui. He was president and minister of the Christian School in Kyoto, Japan. Through his studies of many religions, prayers, and meditations, he realized that a person has to be healed of spirit as well as body. His five principles of life are: today I give thanks for my many blessings; just for today I will not worry; today I will not be angry; today I will do my work honestly; and today I will be kind to my neighbor and to every living thing.

This healing touch is transmitted by the healing touch from a Reiki master to a student. It's that simple. It's the healing power of God that works from within us all that does the work. This is not to be confused with the left brain ego.

I have not only done Reiki on humans but also on animals and plants. I have even used it for difficult situations, such as relationship issues. It can be given not only by adults but also by children and animals.

Just remember, love enough to care and care enough to reach out and touch. When you place your hands on another with the utmost good intentions, beautiful things happen.

In my twenty-three years of having the honor to give and receive Reiki, I have both seen and personally experienced incredible healing. Since I am such an animal lover, here is one of my favorite stories.

A friend of mine who is a Reiki master attuned all her animals to give Reiki. One day while she was barefoot in her home, she stubbed her toe hard on a chair in the living room. She sat in the chair, and her dog came running over and immediately lay on her foot. My friend stayed there for about five minutes. As she stood up to walk, her dog pushed her back into the chair and continued to sit on her foot about ten more minutes. When he felt that she was not accepting the energy anymore, he got up and gave her the OK to move about. She said her foot felt great!

As a human giving Reiki, you can tell when the energy stops flowing through your hands. That says that the receiver has had enough for now. It seems like sweet Petey (the dog) knew, too.

Conclusion

I am here, and I shall not leave you...until you have fulfilled your reason for being.

—Archangel Gabriel

As overwhelming as all of this may seem, I have just barely touched the tip of the iceberg, both of the topics discussed and of the many other options available to you. This book is only the beginning of your journey.

You must be your own best advocate for your health and well-being. Do not completely trust any one person or opinion. Do your research. Most importantly, trust your intuition, and ask to be guided to who or what will help you now in your current situation. Your wishes and prayers are always heard by God and spirit when asked. Trust completely that when the time is right, an answer will be presented to you.

Above all, each of you is unique in every way. You are your very own blueprint to the world. We are all here to serve each other with our gifts and talents. Our spirit needs a physical body to carry out our work to the fullest potential here on Earth. Nourish your body temple, my friends, as it has been asked of us.

Knowledge is power, but wisdom is mastery.

—Laura Walker

Blessings in love and light.

About the Author

Laurie Neri Barrett, registered massage therapist and medical exercise specialist, has been in the fitness health and wellness field since 1986.

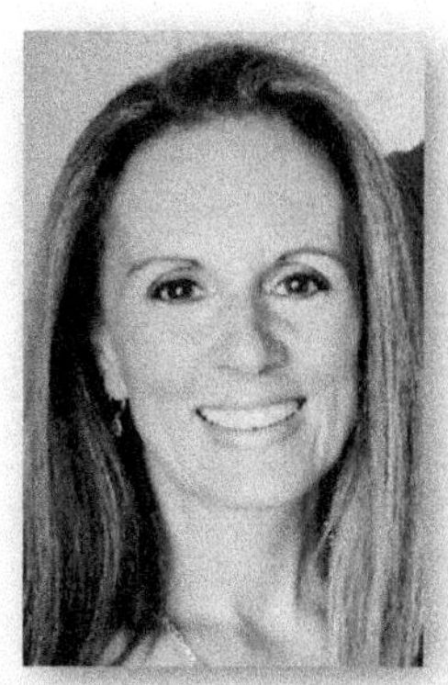

Laurie Neri Barrett

She has worked extensively with all populations. Her background in body therapies—such as Pilates, functional movement, yoga, postinjury rehabilitation, massage, CST, Reiki, and Feldenkrais—brings a unique and individualized focus to the personalized workout. Her accomplishments have been recognized by the National Register's *Who's Who in Executives and Professionals 2006–2007* edition. Her business, Synchronized Kneads, Inc., has also been selected by the US Commerce Association for a Best of Local Business award in the category of outstanding exercise facility for 2010–2011 in addition to her award for Best Pilates for 2013. She was also on staff with the Pilates Institute of London as a certifying teacher in 2006 and 2007.

In addition to working with the human population, Laurie is certified by the Lightfoot Way as an animal consultant. She helps animals and humans bond their relationships by assisting with muscle testing, nutrition, aromatherapy, Bach remedies, homeopathy, crystal and gem remedies, and animal communications.

She continues to educate herself and her staff to have a personal and professional commitment to the various body-mind therapies and overall health and wellness. Laurie is currently continuing her journey by exploring and experiencing the enlightening world of shamanism and energy medicine. Please visit her website at www.synchkneads.com.

References

American Institute for Cancer Research. "Homepage." www.aicr.org.

Anhorn, Nicholas, and Lyndsay Wareham. "Naturopathic by Nature: Healthy Eating and Healthy Living." www.naturopathicbynature.com.

Arnold, Larry, and Sandy Nevius. *The Reiki Handbook: A Manual for Students and Therapists of the Usui Shiki Ryoho System of Healing.* Harrisburg, PA: PSI Press, 1982.

Aston, Judith. *Aston Postural Assessment Workbook: Skills for Observing and Evaluating Body Patterns.* San Antonio, TX: Therapy Skill Builders, 1998.

Breast Cancer Conqueror. "Breast Cancer Conqueror: Empowering Women Around the Globe." www.breastcancerconqueror.com.

Brownstein, David. *Overcoming Thyroid Disorders.* Second Edition. West Bloomfield, MI: Medical Alternative Press, 2008.

Brownstein, David. *The Miracle of Natural Hormones.* Third Edition. West Bloomfield, MI: Medical Alternative Press, 2003.

Cook, Gray. *Movement Functional Movement Systems: Screening, Assessment, and Corrective Strategies.* Aptos, CA: On Target Publications, 2010.

Diamond, John. *Your Body Doesn't Lie: Unlock the Power of Your Natural Energy!* New York, NY: Grand Central Publishing, 1979.

Earth Clinic. Castor Oil. www.earthclinic.com/remedies/castor_oil.html.

Engels-Smith, Jan. *Through the Rabbit Hole.* Seattle, WA: Createspace Independent Publishing Platform, *2014.*

Group, Edward F. *The Green Body Cleanse.* Houston, TX: Global Healing Center, LP, 2010.

Hay, Louise. *You Can Heal Your Life.* Carlsbad, CA: Hay House, Inc., 1999.

Karon, Amy. "Whole Body Cryotherapy Improved Mild Cognitive Impairment in Small Uncontrolled Trial." *Clinical Psychiatry News.* September 20, 2016.

Masiello, Domenick J. "Welcome to My Practice." www.drmasiello.com.

McDonald, Pamela. *The Apo E Gene Diet.* Danville, CA: Prescott Medical Corporation, 2007.

Merck Pharmaceuticals. *The Merck Manual of Diagnosis and Therapy.* Twelfth Edition. Rahway, NJ: Merck Publishing, 1972.

Rao, Preeti. "Integrative Health: A Guide to a Perfect Mind-Body Balance." www.integrativehealthjournal.com.

Reilly, Harold J., and Ruth Hagy Brod. *The Edgar Cayce Handbook for Health: Through Drugless Therapy.* Virginia Beach, VA: ARE Press, 1975.

Reiss, Uzzi. *The Natural Superwoman: The Scientifically Backed Program for Feeling Great, Looking Younger, and Enjoying Amazing Energy at Any Age.* New York, NY: Penguin Group, 2007.

Rose, Jeanne. *The Aromatherapy Book: Applications and Inhalations.* San Francisco, CA: Herbal Studies Course/Jeanne Rose, 1992.

Verstegen, Mark, and Pete Williams. *Core Performance*. Emmaus, PA: Rodale, Inc., 2004.

Weil, Andrew. "What Is Acupuncture?" www.drweil.com/health- wellness/ balanced-living/wellness-therapies/acupuncture/.

9 781978 024632